Your Secret Is

Not

Safe with Me

Corrona Boston, LPC, ATR

&

Nikia Evans

**Illustrations by Ronald Glass III,
Tristen Glass and Zoey Anthony**

Book Design By: Junnita Jackson

Edited By: Nikia Evans

Jacket Design By: Ronald Glass (hand-drawn)
First Edition

Acknowledgements

I want to give a special thank you to my sister Nikia Evans and nephews and niece Ronald Glass III, Tristen Glass and Zoey Anthony for being a part of Auntie's project. It made the experience that much special. Thank you for allowing me to share a piece of my line-of-work and passion with you. Through working together, I hope to have instilled unity, awareness and a sense of accomplishment! In order to build a community, it first starts within your own home. I also want to acknowledge my mother Natalie Boston for showing me the sky is not the limit. To family and friends for their endless affirmations, and above all my Lord and Savior, Jesus Christ for giving me the strength and gifts to help others!

Words of Encouragement from the Illustrator

Ronald C. Glass III- *"If someone threatens you not to tell your parents, still tell them because the abuser is not there with you. The abuser cannot stop you from telling; it's your voice SPEAK UP!"*

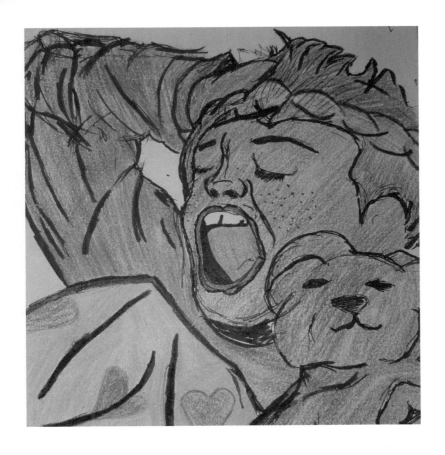

"Rise and shine Tiara!", mommy said, with a warm smile. She leaned in for a loving hug and whispered, "breakfast is ready" as I yarned. The smell of pancakes, turkey bacon and eggs danced across my nose. "Umm", I love the taste of mom's breakfast in the morning. After eating, I grabbed my lunch and it was off to school to learn!

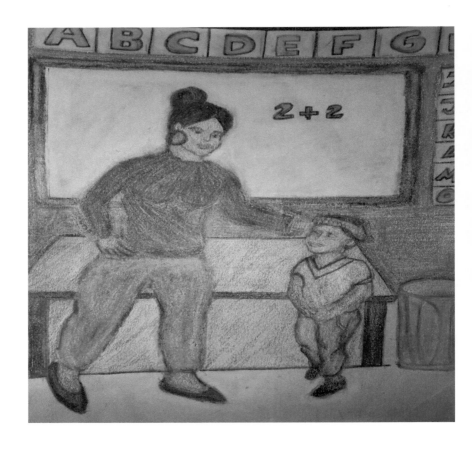

I love Mrs. Flowerton's 2nd grade class. Every day, we learn something new and exciting! Today, we did my favorite; finger painting! I used yellow. I love it so much; it's bright like the sun. Mrs. Flowerton loved it too. She gave me a shiny star sticker; smiled and said, "Tiara, someday you will be a famous artist." I said, "thanks", then the bell rang, and we were off to recess!

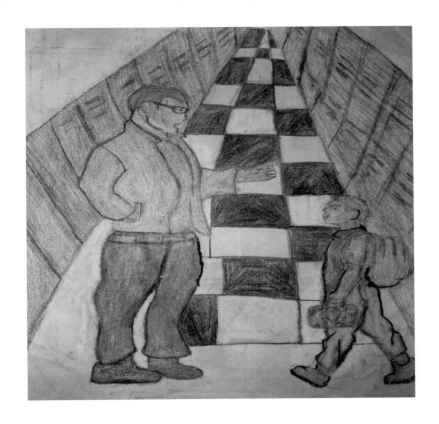

After recess, I was told my mommy was working late again. My neighbor, Mr. Dennis, offered to pick me up from school. After, dismissal he was waiting for me in the hallway. Before leaving, we waved good-bye to Mrs. Flowerton. With her warm smile and pleasant voice, she said, "Tiara, I look forward to seeing you tomorrow." She's the best teacher ever!

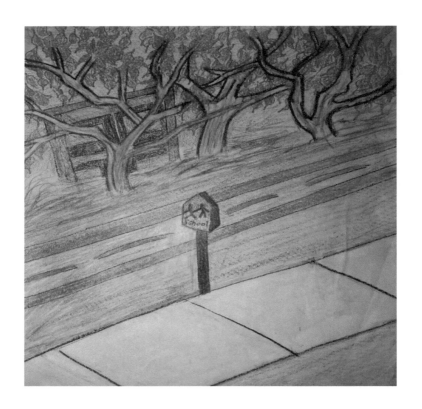

Last time, Mr. Dennis took me straight home and helped me with my homework. But today, he wanted to go to his house first. On the inside, I got a funny feeling in the pit of my stomach. My body did not feel well, but he promised it would be okay. We kept walking as he grabbed my hand.

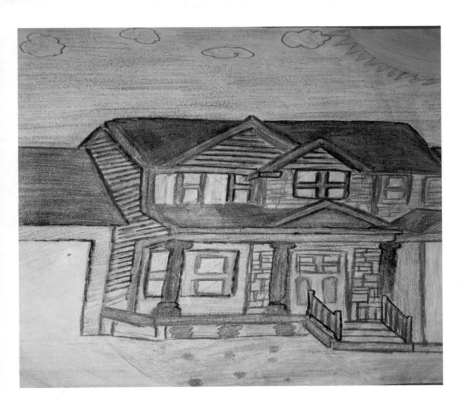

"Tiara, I have a surprise for you today, but it's at my house", Mr. Dennis said. Then he began staring at me through his glasses and asked, "Can you keep a secret?" I nodded my headed as we walked through his hallway, but I was not sure about what was going to happen next. The lights were dim, and the house was still and quiet; as we walked, he promised to be nice if I kept a secret. As we approached his door, I stood there, but not sure of what was going to happen next.

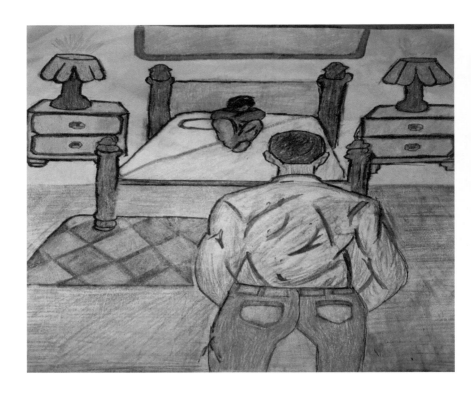

We walked into his bedroom. He gave me a bowl of vanilla ice cream with sprinkles; it's my favorite! Then he started to touch me; I yelled, "no, stop!" He didn't listen. He touched me in a place where mommy says no one ever should. My body and feelings were hurt. I started to cry. He said everything will be okay as long as I kept this a secret. I felt scared, so I said, "yes." Then he took me home.

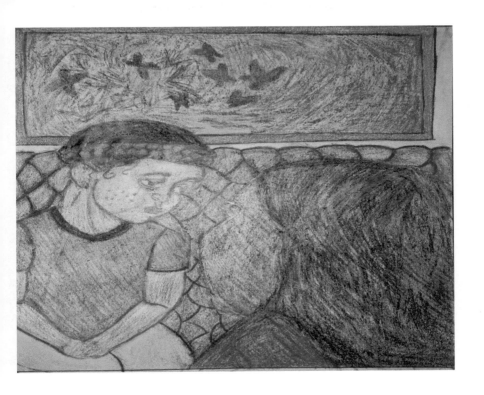

Once I got home, I wanted to say something to my mom, but would she believe me? When she asked about my day, I was afraid if I told on Mr. Dennis, he would hurt me again. I didn't know what to do; so, I told mommy I was tired. I laid in her arms as she held me close and said in her soft sweet voice, "Tiara, everything will be okay." We read a bedtime story and said our prayers. Mommy turned out the light, but I still couldn't sleep. All I could see was the glasses on Mr. Dennis face, in that dim hallway.

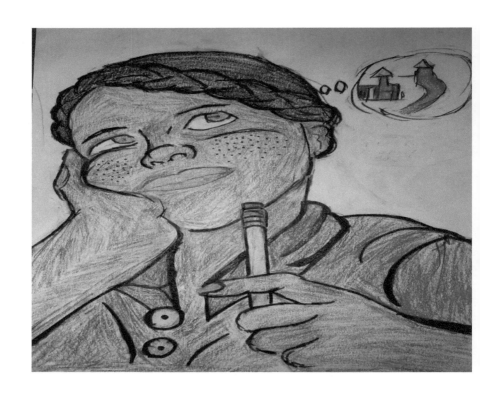

The next morning my alarm rang; it was time for school. I hoped mom's warm hugs and pancakes would make me feel better, but it didn't. I still felt sad and alone. At first it was hard to focus, in school. Then I heard Mrs. Flowerton say, "class, today we are learning about good touch/bad touch; and how to use our voice to say NO!" I also learned it was okay to share bad secrets with someone you trust; like a parent or teacher. I started to feel better.

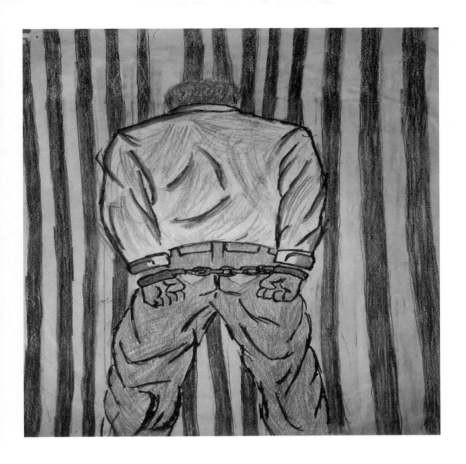

After school, as I was walking to my locker, I saw Mr. Dennis waiting for me. I ran back to Ms. Flowerton, begging her not to let me go with him. I told her all about the bad secret Mr. Dennis asked me to keep. Ms. Flowerton took me to the Counselor and called my mommy. The cops came and took Mr. Dennis away. Now, I know if anyone ever touches me like that again; I will tell someone. From now on those kinds of secrets will never be safe with me!

Appendix

- Normand, Bridgid (2017). Commitment For Children Teaching Touching Safety Rules: Safe and Unsafe Touching.
  https://www.cfchildren.org/blog/2017/08/activity-teaching-touching-safety-rules-safe-and-unsafe-touching/

- Educate 2 Empower Publishing Resource Poster. (2012).https://e2epublishing.info/poster

- Rape Assault Incest National Network (RAINN) Talking to your kids about sexual assault. (2020). https://www.rainn.org/articles/talking-your-kids-about-sexual-assault

- Montgomery County Public School. (2020) Child Abuse and Neglect. www.montgomeryschoolsmd.org

How to Have Uncomfortable Conversations

To Develop Shameless Solutions

Knowing when and how to talk to your child about body safety, can seem nearly impossible. However, being intentional about integrating these types of conversations into a life style routine, can empower your child. This practice will help cultivate education, awareness, support and acquisitional skills necessary to protect your child and keep them safe.

In the book, Your Secret is Not Safe with Me, Tiara have a supportive mother; however, she appears to lack the skills for self-regulating and knowing the proper steps to take after experiencing a traumatic situation. The outcome of her initial response resulted in self-doubt and shame. It was not until Tiara received the education about body safety that she became empowered, and took action that ultimately led to an arrest and prevention of another sexual assault.

Being a child that is the victim of trauma can have a devastating impact on their psychological and physical wellness. Therefore, it is imperative to know that if shame is the root of a problem; then shame can never be a part of the solution that leads to recovery. Whether exposed to a one-time traumatic event, or several years of intergenerational trauma; the child must feel safe in order to remove the power of secrecy by sharing their story. Secrecy holds power that can cause the child to isolate and perpetuate an endless cycle of re-experiencing that trauma. To break the cycle and change the trajectory of the child's life; it is important to provide a platform where their voices can be heard; that they may be able to move beyond their trauma.

Below is an informative chart that describes the different styles of communication; and how it can impact individuals during a dialogue; along with conversation starter tips about body safety.

Healthy and Effective Communication Tools

The Outcome	Passive	Aggressive	Passive/ Aggressive	Assertive
Behavior: *(How this looks when put into action i.e. verbally or nonverbally)*	Chooses not to express feelings or needs, prioritize needs of others, lacks self-confidence, timid tone and allows others to take advantage	Dominate others, interrupts frequently, impulsive, dismissive, and blame others	Difficulties acknowledging one's own anger, deny problem exists, indirect hostility and uses sarcasm to minimize real feelings	Clearly, fairly and directly state one's own needs, intentionally communicate respectfully and empathetically, relaxed body posture and calm tone
The Impact: *(The direct result of how the chosen style of*	Feels resentful/ unfairly treated, which could result in becoming	Always blame/never take ownership-making it difficult to mature,	Remain unheard and powerless	Feel connected to others

15

communication influences Emotions)	depressed or anxious	causes fear or dislike by others		
Beliefs: *(Ideas that helps interprets everyday reality)*	No one will ever consider my feelings	One is always right, and One can violate others	One will appear like he/she agrees and is cooperative, but is not	Confident, understand choices are available, and the only person one can control is oneself

Ways to Prevent an Argument when Having Uncomfortable Conversations:

When creating a safe place for healthy communication about uncomfortable topics please remember your tone, body language and choice of words. Remaining calm and warm can help put the victim of sexual assault at ease, and possibly determine the degree of information shared:

- **Actively listen before interrupting-** "So tell me what you think the rules are for keeping your body parts safe?"
- **Prioritize finding agreement and one's personal experiences over technicality, and your own truth or beliefs-** "It's normal to feel nervous or uncomfortable when I ask you about touch. But I want you to know I am here to listen as you tell me more about what happened next from your view."
- **Know when and how to make an INTENTIONAL effort to help one with feeling safe and supported-** "You are brave, and safe now. You have a voice that is heard. Let me know what support looks like, so I can help."
- **Don't jump to conclusions-** "I don't want to say what I think happened, so it's important to tell me what you remember."
- **Be willing to change, compromise and communicate when needed-** "You did the right thing coming to me. I know you shared a lot, so if you need a break I understand. We can talk later."

Body Safety

When communicating about body safety, it is important to be aware of the basic keywords, commands, and actual body parts to help educate your child on their rights. Below are various ways to address these topics.

First steps for identifying body safety:

- Identify which areas of their body are private
- Identify whether a touch is "safe" or "unsafe/unwanted
- Recognize how to avoid and refuse unsafe/unwanted touches
- Identify the difference between good/happy and bad/unsafe secrets
- Identify adults that your child can trust to talk to about any uncomfortable/unsafe things
- Identify ways to tell a trusted adult even when feeling uncomfortable
- Understand that sexual abusers may use tricks, bribes, or threats to gain and maintain trust and secrecy
- Recognize and report child abuse

Various Kind of Touches

Safe Touch	Unsafe Touch	Unwanted Touch
These are touches that keep children safe and are good for them, and that make them feel cared for and important.	These are touches that hurt your body or feelings such as hitting, pushing, pinching, and kicking.	These are touches that might be safe, but a child still does not want from that person or at that moment. It's okay for a child to say no to an unwanted touch, even if it's from a familiar person.
Safe touches can include hugging, pat on the back, and an arm around the shoulder	Touches that hurt your body in private or covered areas.	Help your child practice saying no in a strong, yet polite voice. This will help them learn to set personal boundaries.
Safe touches can also include touches that might hurt, such as removing a splinter. When you remove a splinter, you're doing so to keep them healthy, which makes it a safe touch	Allowing others to touch their body parts in front of you.	Understanding the importance of not safely touching others without asking for permission.

Many children experience internal and external warning signs caused by triggers. By educating them about their bodily responses they will have a language for articulating their experiences.

Body Chart

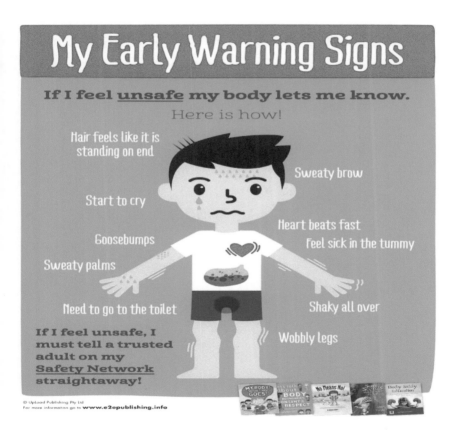

Resources

- Child and Family Services Agency. Report Suspected Child Abuse in DC: (202) 671- SAFE
- Child Welfare Services 24-hrs Hotline: (240) 777- 4417
- Children and Adolescents Mobile Psychiatric Services: (202) 481-1440
- Crime Victims Compensation Program: (202) 879-4216
- RAINN National Number to Reach Counselors Anywhere in the Country: 1-800 656-HOPE ext 4673
- Youth and Preventive Services Division Investigates Cases Involving Minors: (202) 576-6768

About the Author:

Corrona serves the District of Columbia communities as a passionate Psychotherapist, Art Therapist, and Creative Freelancer. She operates as the owner of ArtVersity, birthed from the belief each person has a God-given gift that enables them to produce something great. She is a native of the urban communities of Baltimore City, and was introduced to the arts by her father. Corrona states, "ArtVersity started because my dad recognized something in me, which I overlooked. Now I want to provide individuals' an opportunity to see aspects of themselves that typically go unnoticed, and bring it out in order for them to become inspired".

Her passion to understand the creative arts using various applications led to matriculation at Drexel University earning her M A. in Creative Arts in Therapy. She received the opportunity to work for several mental health agencies in the surrounding DMV area such as Johns Hopkins Hospital, school-based settings and mental health organizations servicing at-risk populations. Her extensive educational and professional background in both traditional and expressive art therapies is a unique asset for the serving population. Her clinical experience includes traditional theoretical approaches, in addition to evidenced-based models including Trauma Systems Therapy and MultiSystemic Therapy. Additionally, Corrona received the honor to serve as a Guest Speaker to address Mental Health, Art Therapy and Healthy Relationships concerns at Howard University, Bowie State University and Coppin State University.

Corrona's style of therapy promotes empowerment and personal insight into oneself through expressive arts. With this specialty, she seized the opportunity to create and co-develop her first silent art auction, called, "Artist in Me ". This opened the door for her to continue flourishing in her craft by facilitating Sip N' Paints for schools, organizations and home-based clients, and providing counseling, art therapy and workshops services. ArtVersity encourages clients to embrace the diversity of the arts and integrate it into everyday life without limits.

For more information about Corrona and services provided, please visit her website at www.corronaboston.com

About the Author:

Mrs. Nikia Evans, a novice writer and native of Baltimore City; is an alumnus of Howard University, with over 15 years of experience as an arts education professional. She is a wife and mother of six beautiful children; including the principal illustrator of this publication, Ronald Glass III (age 12) and the contributing illustrators of this book, Zoey Anthony (age 10) and Tristen Glass (age 11). Mrs. Evans enjoys working with children; composing music; writing poetry; plays; and short stories.